Ultimate Weight Loss Handbook: 500 Tips to Transform Your Body and Life

MARTIN STEVENS

ISBN: 9798880034482

DEDICATION

This book is dedicated to:

To my family, whose unwavering support and encouragement have been the cornerstone of this journey. Your love and belief in me have been my greatest motivation.

To my friends, for being my source of inspiration and laughter, and for sharing in the joys and challenges of life.

To the countless individuals who shared their stories, struggles, and triumphs—your experiences have shaped the heart of this book.

And to every reader embarking on their own path to wellness. May these pages offer guidance, inspiration, and the tools to transform your body and life.

With heartfelt appreciation,

Martin Stevens

TABLE OF CONTENTS

Chapter 6: Special Considerations

Chapter 7: Supplement and Lifestyle Enhancements

Chapter 8: Conclusion

Ultimate Weight Loss Handbook:
500 Tips to Transform Your Body and Life

Appendix A: Sample Meal Plans

Appendix B: Workout Routine Templates

Appendix C: Food and Exercise Journal Template

Appendix D: Glossary of Terms

Ultimate Weight Loss Handbook:
500 Tips to Transform Your Body and Life

ACKNOWLEDGMENTS

I would like to express my deepest gratitude to everyone who contributed to the creation of this comprehensive weight loss handbook. Writing this book would not have been possible without the support, expertise, and encouragement of many individuals.

A special thank you goes to the nutritionists, fitness experts, and health professionals who generously shared their knowledge and insights. Your expertise has added credibility and depth to the tips and advice presented in this handbook.

I extend my appreciation to the beta readers and volunteers who provided valuable feedback during the development stages. Your input has been crucial in refining the content and ensuring its relevance and accessibility to a wide audience.

To my friends and family, thank you for your constant support and understanding during the long hours spent researching and writing. Your encouragement has been a source of inspiration throughout this journey.

Lastly, I want to express my gratitude to the readers who choose to embark on this weight loss journey with the help of this handbook. Your commitment to improving your health and well-being is commendable, and I hope this resource proves to be a valuable companion on your path to a healthier lifestyle.

Thank you all for being a part of this project and contributing to its success.

"Your body is a reflection of your lifestyle choices. Transform it with purpose, nourish it with wisdom, and sculpt it with determination." - Anonymous

Legal Disclaimer:

Please note that the information provided in this book is for informational purposes only and should not be considered as professional advice. Readers are encouraged to consult with relevant experts or professionals for personalized guidance.

Ultimate Weight Loss Handbook:
500 Tips to Transform Your Body and Life

PREFACE

Welcome to the "Ultimate Weight Loss Handbook: 500 Tips to Transform Your Body and Life." This comprehensive guide is designed to be your go-to resource on the journey towards achieving a healthier, more fulfilling lifestyle. Whether you're just starting on your weight loss journey or seeking to fine-tune your existing practices, this handbook is here to empower and guide you.

In a world inundated with fad diets, conflicting fitness advice, and quick fixes, it's essential to have a reliable source that distills evidence-based information into practical tips. The tips provided in this handbook are not just about shedding pounds but about embracing a holistic approach to wellness. We believe in empowering you to make sustainable lifestyle changes that promote long-term health and happiness.

This handbook is structured to cover various aspects of weight loss, from understanding the fundamentals of nutrition and exercise to addressing the mental and emotional aspects that often accompany this transformative journey. The tips presented here are not one-size-fits-all; instead, they are a diverse collection to cater to different preferences, lifestyles, and circumstances.

As you embark on this journey, remember that change is a gradual process, and small, consistent efforts can lead to significant transformations. This handbook is not a strict rule book but a guide to help you navigate the complexities of weight loss with confidence and clarity.

We encourage you to approach the tips with an open mind, experiment with what works best for you, and celebrate the progress you make along the way. Your journey is unique, and this handbook is here to support you every step of the way.

Here's to your health, happiness, and the transformative power within you.

Best wishes,

Martin Stevens

Author, "Ultimate Weight Loss Handbook"

Ultimate Weight Loss Handbook:
500 Tips to Transform Your Body and Life

FOREWORD

In the landscape of health and fitness, finding trustworthy guidance can be a daunting task. Amidst the noise of conflicting advice and quick fixes, the "Ultimate Weight Loss Handbook: 500 Tips to Transform Your Body and Life" emerges as a beacon of clarity and practical wisdom.

We all witness firsthand the struggles individuals face on their weight loss journeys. This handbook, penned by Martin Stevens, is a remarkable compilation of evidence-based tips that cut through the confusion, offering a roadmap for those seeking sustainable and meaningful change.

What sets this handbook apart is its holistic approach. It goes beyond mere numbers on a scale, delving into the interconnected realms of nutrition, exercise, mental well-being, and lifestyle choices. The author emphasizes the importance of balance, mindfulness, and realistic goal setting, recognizing that true transformation involves both the body and the mind.

The tips presented here are not rigid prescriptions but versatile tools, adaptable to various lifestyles and preferences. Each tip is grounded in a commitment to long-term health, encouraging readers to cultivate habits that stand the test of time.

You'll find a wealth of knowledge from experts in nutrition, fitness, and well-being. The handbook is not just about shedding pounds; it's about fostering a positive relationship with your body, nurturing it with care, and embracing the journey towards a healthier, happier you.

PROLOGUE

In the pursuit of weight loss, we often find ourselves at the crossroads of desire and determination, seeking a path that leads not only to a lighter physical self but also to a fuller, more vibrant life. The journey is deeply personal, marked by challenges, triumphs, and a myriad of emotions.

The "Ultimate Weight Loss Handbook" is more than just a compilation of tips; it is an invitation to embark on a transformative voyage. In this prologue, we set the stage for the exploration of not just the body but the intricate interplay of mind, spirit, and lifestyle choices.

As we delve into the 500 tips curated by Martin Stevens, remember that this is not a rigid prescription but a versatile toolkit. Each tip is a steppingstone, guiding you toward a healthier, more balanced existence. This handbook is not about quick fixes or temporary solutions; it is a commitment to lasting change.

The prologue serves as a moment of reflection—a pause to consider the motivations that brought you to this point and the aspirations that propel you forward. It is an acknowledgment that transformation is not solely about shedding pounds but about redefining your relationship with yourself, your habits, and your environment.

Through these pages, you will encounter a wealth of insights, practical advice, and the collective wisdom of experts in nutrition, fitness, and well-being. The journey ahead is both challenging and rewarding, and this prologue invites you to embrace it with an open heart and a resilient spirit.

Ultimate Weight Loss Handbook:
500 Tips to Transform Your Body and Life

Introduction:

Welcome to the "Ultimate Weight Loss Handbook: 500 Tips to Transform Your Body and Life." In a world where health and wellness are paramount, this handbook serves as your comprehensive guide to achieving sustainable weight loss and embracing a healthier lifestyle.

0.1 Why Weight Loss Matters:

Beyond the aesthetics, weight loss holds profound implications for your overall well-being. This section explores the multifaceted reasons why embarking on a weight loss journey is a meaningful and transformative endeavor. From improving physical health to enhancing mental and emotional resilience, understanding the significance of this journey is the first step toward lasting change.

0.2 Setting Realistic Goals:

Effective goal-setting is the bedrock of any successful weight loss journey. Here, we delve into the art of setting realistic and achievable goals tailored to your unique circumstances.

By aligning your aspirations with practical objectives, you pave the way for a journey that is both rewarding and sustainable.

0.3 Understanding the Basics of Weight Loss:

Before embarking on the 500 tips detailed in this handbook, it's essential to grasp the fundamentals of weight loss. This section provides an overview of the key components, including the role of nutrition, exercise, and lifestyle choices. Building a solid foundation of understanding ensures that you approach your journey with informed decisions and confidence.

As you navigate the pages of this handbook, keep in mind that your journey is a personal one. The 500 tips offered here are not a rigid roadmap but rather a versatile toolkit, allowing you to tailor your approach to fit your lifestyle, preferences, and individual needs. Whether you are just beginning your weight loss journey or seeking to refine your existing practices, this handbook is designed to empower and guide you toward a healthier, more fulfilling life.

Let the transformation begin.

Chapter 1: Nutrition Tips

In the pursuit of weight loss, what you eat plays a pivotal role in shaping your journey. This chapter delves into the intricacies of nutrition, offering practical tips to guide you toward a balanced and sustainable diet.

1.1 Balanced Diet Essentials:

Embark on your weight loss journey by understanding the essentials of a balanced diet. Explore the benefits of incorporating a variety of nutrient-dense foods into your meals, emphasizing the importance of fruits, vegetables, lean proteins, whole grains, and healthy fats. Discover how a colorful plate can not only aid in weight management but also contribute to overall well-being.

1.2 Portion Control Strategies:

Effective weight management often hinges on portion control. Learn practical strategies to avoid overeating, tune in to your body's hunger and fullness cues, and foster mindful eating habits. Discover that enjoying your favorite foods is possible while still maintaining a healthy balance.

1.3 The Role of Macronutrients:

Uncover the significance of macronutrients—carbohydrates, proteins, and fats—in achieving your weight loss goals. Delve into the nuanced roles each macronutrient plays in fueling your body, promoting muscle growth, and supporting overall health. Learn to strike the right balance that aligns with your individual needs.

1.4 Smart Snacking Ideas:

Snacking can be both satisfying and supportive of your weight loss journey when approached mindfully. Explore nutritious and delicious snack options that keep you energized between meals. From protein-packed snacks to fiber-rich options, discover how smart snacking can contribute to your overall nutritional goals.

1.5 Hydration for Weight Loss:

Proper hydration is often underestimated in its impact on weight loss. Gain insights into the benefits of staying well-hydrated, understand how hydration affects metabolism, and learn practical tips to ensure you meet your daily fluid needs. Discover the subtle yet transformative role water plays in your overall well-being.

As you navigate the nutritional aspects outlined in this chapter, remember that sustainable change is built on gradual adjustments and mindful choices. By incorporating these nutrition tips into your daily routine, you're laying the groundwork for a healthier and more nourished version of yourself.

Chapter 2: Exercise and Fitness

Embarking on a holistic weight loss journey involves more than just dietary adjustments; integrating regular physical activity is crucial for achieving lasting results. In this chapter, we delve into the realm of exercise and fitness, providing insights and practical tips to help you craft a well-rounded and effective workout routine.

2.1 Developing a Workout Routine:

Creating a personalized workout routine is the foundation of your fitness journey. Explore the components of a well-balanced exercise plan, incorporating elements of cardiovascular workouts, strength training, and flexibility exercises. Discover the importance of setting realistic goals and progressively increasing the intensity of your workouts to promote overall fitness.

2.2 Cardiovascular Exercises for Fat Burning:

Cardiovascular exercises are instrumental in burning calories and improving cardiovascular health. Delve into a variety of cardio activities, from brisk walking and jogging to cycling and swimming. Understand how these exercises contribute to fat burning, enhance endurance, and support your weight loss goals. Find joy in activities that elevate your heart rate and boost overall well-being.

2.3 Strength Training for a Lean Body:

Building lean muscle mass is key to boosting metabolism and achieving a sculpted physique. Explore the benefits of strength training through various modalities, including weightlifting, bodyweight exercises, and resistance training. Learn how to design a balanced strength training routine that targets different muscle groups, fostering both strength and definition.

2.4 Incorporating High-Intensity Interval Training (HIIT):

High-Intensity Interval Training (HIIT) is a time-efficient and effective approach to fitness. Uncover the principles behind HIIT, which involves alternating between short bursts of intense activity and periods of rest or lower intensity. Discover how HIIT can enhance calorie burning, improve cardiovascular fitness, and provide versatility in your workout routine.

2.5 Flexibility and Core Workouts:

Flexibility and core strength are often overlooked aspects of fitness that contribute to overall well-being. Explore the importance of incorporating stretching and flexibility exercises into your routine for improved mobility and injury prevention. Additionally, delve into core-strengthening exercises that not only support weight loss but also enhance stability and posture.

As you embrace the exercise and fitness tips in this chapter, remember that consistency and variety are key. Choose activities that align with your preferences, mix up your routine to prevent monotony, and celebrate the progress you make on your journey to a healthier, more active lifestyle.

Chapter 3: Mental and Emotional Well-being

Embarking on a weight loss journey is not solely about transforming your body; it also involves nurturing your mental and emotional well-being. In this chapter, we explore the vital connection between your mind and body, providing guidance on cultivating mindfulness, managing stress, prioritizing quality sleep, building a positive body image, and overcoming emotional eating.

3.1 Mindful Eating Practices:

Mindful eating involves being fully present during meals, fostering a deeper connection with your food. Discover techniques that encourage a mindful approach to eating, such as savoring each bite, paying attention to hunger and fullness cues, and avoiding distractions. Learn how cultivating mindfulness can transform your relationship with food and contribute to your weight loss journey.

3.2 Managing Stress and Cortisol Levels:

Stress can impact both your mental well-being and weight. Explore effective stress management techniques to keep cortisol levels in check. From deep breathing exercises and meditation to incorporating relaxation practices into your daily routine, discover how to mitigate stress and its potential impact on weight gain. Embracing stress management strategies contributes not only to your weight loss goals but also to overall health.

3.3 Getting Quality Sleep for Weight Loss:

Quality sleep is a cornerstone of overall well-being and can significantly influence your weight loss journey. Understand the intricate relationship between sleep and metabolism and explore practical tips for improving sleep hygiene. Establishing consistent sleep routines and prioritizing restful sleep not only supports your weight loss efforts but also enhances your overall vitality.

3.4 Building a Positive Body Image:

Cultivating a positive body image is essential for a healthy mindset on your weight loss journey. Challenge societal standards, embrace your unique features, and learn to appreciate your body for its strength and resilience. This section provides insights and exercises to foster self-love and acceptance, recognizing that a positive body image is integral to lasting well-being.

3.5 Overcoming Emotional Eating:

Many individuals turn to food as a way to cope with emotions, such as stress, sadness, or boredom. Uncover strategies to identify and address emotional eating patterns. Learn to distinguish between physical hunger and emotional triggers and explore alternative ways to manage emotions without turning to food. By addressing emotional eating, you empower yourself to make choices that align with your health and wellness goals.

As you navigate the mental and emotional aspects of your weight loss journey, remember that your mindset is a powerful tool. The tips in this chapter aim to guide you toward a balanced and positive relationship with yourself, supporting not only your physical transformation but also your overall well-being.

Chapter 4: Lifestyle Changes

Creating a sustainable and healthy lifestyle is fundamental to the success of your weight loss journey. In this chapter, we explore practical tips for seamlessly integrating physical activity into your daily life, adopting healthy cooking and meal prep habits, making informed choices when dining out, seeking social support, and avoiding common pitfalls that may hinder your progress.

4.1 Incorporating Physical Activity Into Daily Life:

Physical activity is not limited to structured workout sessions. Discover creative ways to infuse movement into your daily routine, such as taking the stairs, walking during breaks, or engaging in active hobbies. These small, consistent efforts contribute to overall physical well-being and support your weight loss goals in the long run.

4.2 Healthy Cooking and Meal Prep Tips:

The choices you make in the kitchen play a pivotal role in your weight loss journey. Explore healthy cooking techniques, ingredient substitutions, and time-saving meal prep strategies. By preparing nutritious meals in advance, you empower yourself to make mindful choices and avoid succumbing to unhealthy options when time is limited.

4.3 Making Informed Food Choices at Restaurants:

Eating out doesn't have to derail your weight loss efforts. Learn how to navigate restaurant menus, make healthier choices when dining out, and practice portion control in social settings. By making informed decisions and being mindful of your choices, you can enjoy meals outside the home without compromising your goals.

4.4 Social Support and Accountability:

Having a support system is invaluable on your weight loss journey. Cultivate social support from friends, family, or online communities to share experiences, challenges, and successes. Explore the benefits of accountability partners and the motivation that comes from knowing you're not alone in your pursuit of a healthier lifestyle.

4.5 Avoiding Common Weight Loss Pitfalls:

Recognizing and addressing common pitfalls is crucial for sustained success. This section highlights potential challenges, such as setting unrealistic expectations, succumbing to emotional eating triggers, and navigating social and environmental factors. Arm yourself with strategies to overcome these obstacles and stay on course toward your weight loss goals.

As you delve into the lifestyle changes outlined in this chapter, remember that building a healthy lifestyle is a gradual process. By incorporating these tips into your daily routine, you're not only supporting your weight loss journey but also laying the foundation for long-term well-being.

Chapter 5: Sustainable Habits for Long-Term Success

Achieving lasting weight loss goes beyond short-term fixes; it involves cultivating sustainable habits that become an integral part of your lifestyle. In this chapter, we explore the importance of creating healthy habits, effective ways to track your progress, strategies for celebrating milestones and rewards, navigating plateaus and challenges, and implementing maintenance strategies for ongoing weight management.

5.1 Creating Healthy Habits That Last:

Establishing healthy habits is the key to long-term success on your weight loss journey. Explore practical tips for incorporating sustainable changes into your daily routine, focusing on nutrition, exercise, sleep, and stress management. By building positive habits, you create a foundation for ongoing well-being.

5.2 Tracking Progress Effectively:

Monitoring your progress is crucial for staying on track and making informed adjustments. Learn about effective tracking methods, from keeping a food and exercise journal to using technology and apps that help monitor your goals. By understanding and analyzing your progress, you empower yourself to make informed decisions on your wellness journey.

5.3 Celebrating Milestones and Rewards:

Acknowledging your achievements is an essential aspect of maintaining motivation. Explore the importance of setting milestones and establishing rewards for reaching them. Discover how celebrating your successes, whether big or small, contributes to a positive mindset and reinforces your commitment to long-term well-being.

5.4 Adapting to Plateaus and Challenges:

Plateaus and challenges are a natural part of any transformative journey. Understand common reasons for plateaus and learn strategies to overcome them. Explore effective ways to navigate challenges, whether they stem from changes in routine, emotional triggers, or external factors. By adapting to setbacks, you can maintain resilience and continue progressing toward your goals.

5.5 Maintenance Strategies for Weight Management:

Sustaining your achievements requires ongoing effort and mindful management. Delve into effective maintenance strategies, including regular reassessment of goals, staying connected with your support system, and adjusting your plan to align with changing circumstances. By adopting a maintenance mindset, you create a framework for lifelong well-being.

As you delve into the sustainable habits outlined in this chapter, remember that your weight loss journey is an ongoing process. By embracing these strategies and incorporating them into your lifestyle, you're not only achieving weight loss but also fostering a healthier and more balanced life.

Chapter 6: Special Considerations

Recognizing the diversity of individual experiences, this chapter addresses specific considerations that may impact weight loss based on age, gender, life stages, and potential medical conditions. Tailoring your approach to these unique factors ensures a more personalized and effective weight loss journey.

6.1 Weight Loss for Different Age Groups:

Age can influence metabolism, activity levels, and nutritional needs. Explore age-specific considerations for weight loss, whether you're a young adult, in midlife, or navigating the challenges and opportunities that come with aging. Understanding how age impacts your body allows for a more targeted and effective approach to your wellness goals.

6.2 Weight Loss During Pregnancy and Postpartum:

Pregnancy and postpartum periods introduce unique considerations for weight management. Discover safe and healthy approaches to weight loss during and after pregnancy, emphasizing the importance of nourishing both yourself and your baby. Explore exercises suitable for different stages and learn about the balance between self-care and the demands of parenthood.

6.3 Addressing Medical Conditions and Medications:

Certain medical conditions and medications can influence weight and complicate weight loss efforts. This section explores considerations for managing weight in the presence of conditions such as thyroid disorders, diabetes, and others. Additionally, understand how medications may impact your weight and strategies for mitigating their effects on your wellness journey.

6.4 Weight Loss for Men vs. Women:

Men and women may experience weight loss differently due to hormonal variations and metabolic differences. Uncover gender-specific considerations and strategies tailored to optimize weight loss for both men and women. Understanding these nuances allows for a more targeted and effective approach based on individual needs.

6.5 Navigating Weight Loss Plateaus:

Weight loss plateaus are common but can be challenging to overcome. Explore strategies to break through plateaus, whether they're due to changes in metabolism, adjustments in your routine, or psychological factors. Learn how to adapt your approach, reassess goals, and stay motivated during these temporary lulls in progress.

Navigating these special considerations ensures a more holistic and personalized approach to your weight loss journey. By addressing factors specific to your age, gender, health conditions, and potential plateaus, you empower yourself to make informed decisions that align with your unique circumstances.

Chapter 7: Supplement and Lifestyle Enhancements

In this chapter, we explore the role of supplements, vitamins, and lifestyle enhancements that can complement your weight loss journey. While no substitute for a healthy diet and regular exercise, these elements can play a supportive role in optimizing your overall well-being.

7.1 Understanding Weight Loss Supplements:

Explore the world of weight loss supplements, understanding their potential benefits and limitations. Learn about commonly used supplements, such as those containing caffeine, green tea extract, or fiber. Discover the importance of cautious supplementation, with an emphasis on transparency, research, and consulting with healthcare professionals before incorporating any supplements into your routine.

7.2 The Role of Vitamins and Minerals:

Vitamins and minerals are essential for various bodily functions, and deficiencies can impact your overall health. Delve into the role of key vitamins and minerals in supporting weight loss and metabolism. Explore food sources rich in these nutrients and learn about the potential benefits of supplementation, keeping in mind that a balanced diet is the primary source of essential nutrients.

7.3 Integrating Detoxification Practices:

Detoxification practices have gained popularity in the wellness sphere. Understand the principles behind detoxification, explore safe and evidence-based methods, and learn how these practices may support your weight loss goals. Emphasize holistic approaches that focus on nourishing your body and eliminating harmful substances.

7.4 Stress Reduction Techniques:

Chronic stress can hinder weight loss efforts. Explore stress reduction techniques such as meditation, deep breathing exercises, yoga, and mindfulness practices. By incorporating stress management into your routine, you can positively impact your mental and physical well-being, creating a more conducive environment for weight loss.

7.5 Mind-Body Practices for Weight Loss:

Mind-body practices, including activities like meditation, tai chi, and yoga, can contribute to a balanced and holistic approach to weight loss. Discover how these practices promote self-awareness, mindfulness, and a positive mindset. Embrace the mind-body connection as a valuable component of your weight loss journey.

As you explore supplement and lifestyle enhancements, remember that these elements are meant to complement, not replace, a healthy diet and regular exercise. Before making significant changes to your routine, consult with healthcare professionals to ensure that these strategies align with your individual needs and health status.

Chapter 8: Conclusion

Congratulations on reaching the final chapter of the "Ultimate Weight Loss Handbook: 500 Tips to Transform Your Body and Life." This chapter serves as a culmination of the insights and strategies presented throughout the book, providing a comprehensive summary and offering guidance as you move forward on your transformative journey.

8.1 Recap of Key Takeaways:

Reflect on the key takeaways from each chapter, emphasizing the foundational principles that contribute to successful weight loss. Recap the importance of balanced nutrition, regular exercise, mindfulness, and the adoption of sustainable lifestyle habits. Revisit the tips that resonated most with you and consider how they have influenced your approach to health and wellness.

8.2 Encouragement for the Journey Ahead:

Embarking on a weight loss journey requires dedication, resilience, and a positive mindset. Take a moment to acknowledge your progress, no matter how small, and recognize the effort you've invested in your well-being. Embrace the journey as a continuous process of growth, learning, and self-discovery.

8.3 Resources and Further Reading:

To support your ongoing commitment to health, this section provides additional resources and recommended readings. Explore reputable sources, websites, and books that delve deeper into specific topics related to nutrition, exercise, mental well-being, and lifestyle changes. Continuously educating yourself ensures that you stay informed and empowered on your journey.

As you conclude this handbook, remember that transformation is a dynamic and individualized process. Your journey is unique, and there is no one-size-fits-all approach to weight loss. Embrace the lessons learned, celebrate your successes, and remain adaptable to the evolving needs of your body and mind.

The "Ultimate Weight Loss Handbook" is more than a guide; it is a companion on your path to a healthier and more fulfilling life. May your journey be filled with resilience, self-discovery, and the joy of achieving lasting well-being.

Wishing you continued success and vibrant health,

Martin Stevens

Author, "Ultimate Weight Loss Handbook"

Appendix A: Sample Meal Plans

In this appendix, you'll find a collection of sample meal plans designed to provide inspiration and guidance for creating balanced, nutritious, and satisfying meals. These plans incorporate a variety of food options, emphasizing portion control, essential nutrients, and diverse flavors. Remember that these are examples, and you can customize them based on your preferences, dietary restrictions, and nutritional needs.

Sample Meal Plan 1:

- Breakfast: Greek yogurt with mixed berries and a sprinkle of chia seeds

- Snack: Apple slices with almond butter

- Lunch: Grilled chicken salad with mixed greens, cherry tomatoes, cucumbers, and vinaigrette dressing

- Snack: Hummus with carrot and celery sticks

- Dinner: Baked salmon, quinoa, and roasted vegetables (broccoli, bell peppers, and zucchini)

Sample Meal Plan 2:

- Breakfast: Oatmeal with banana slices, walnuts, and a drizzle of honey

- Snack: Cottage cheese with pineapple chunks

- Lunch: Whole grain wrap with turkey, avocado, lettuce, and tomato

- Snack: Greek yogurt parfait with granola and mixed berries

- Dinner: Stir-fried tofu with brown rice and a medley of colorful vegetables (bell peppers, snap peas, and carrots)

Sample Meal Plan 3:

- Breakfast: Scrambled eggs with spinach and whole-grain toast

- Snack: Mixed nuts (almonds, walnuts, and pistachios)

- Lunch: Quinoa salad with chickpeas, feta cheese, cherry tomatoes, and a lemon-tahini dressing

- Snack: Orange slices with a handful of almonds

- Dinner: Grilled shrimp skewers, sweet potato wedges, and steamed broccoli

Feel free to use these sample meal plans as a starting point for creating your own, keeping in mind the importance of variety, balance, and moderation in your dietary choices. Consult with a healthcare professional or nutritionist to ensure that your meal plans align with your individual nutritional needs and health goals.

Appendix B: Workout Routine Templates

In this appendix, you'll find workout routine templates to assist you in structuring effective and diverse exercise plans. These templates cater to different fitness levels and preferences, offering flexibility for customization based on your individual goals and time constraints. Before starting any new exercise regimen, consult with a fitness professional or healthcare provider to ensure it aligns with your fitness level and health status.

Workout Routine Template 1: Beginner's Full-Body Workout

1. Warm-up (5-10 minutes):

   - Light cardio (e.g., jogging in place or jumping jacks)

   - Dynamic stretches (arm circles, leg swings)

2. Strength Training (20-30 minutes):

   - Bodyweight squats: 3 sets of 12 reps

   - Push-ups: 3 sets of 10 reps

   - Bent-over rows (using water bottles or light weights): 3 sets of 12 reps per arm

   - Plank: 3 sets, holding for 30 seconds to 1 minute

3. Cardio (15-20 minutes):

   - Brisk walking, cycling, or dancing

4. Cool Down (5-10 minutes):

- Static stretches targeting major muscle groups

- Deep breathing or meditation

**Workout Routine Template 2:
Intermediate Split Routine**

1. Warm-up (10 minutes):

   - Jump rope or brisk walking

   - Dynamic stretches

2. Strength Training (40 minutes):

   - Monday (Upper Body): Bench press, pull-ups, dumbbell curls, triceps dips

   - Wednesday (Lower Body): Squats, lunges, leg press, calf raises

   - Friday (Core): Plank variations, Russian twists, bicycle crunches

3. Cardio and HIIT (15-20 minutes):

   - Interval training, alternating between high-intensity bursts and recovery periods

4. Cool Down (10 minutes):

   - Static stretches for each muscle group

   - Deep breathing exercises

**Workout Routine Template 3:
Advanced Full-Body Circuit**

Perform each exercise for 45 seconds, followed by a 15-second rest. Complete the circuit 3 times.

1. Burpees

2. Mountain climbers

3. Kettlebell swings

4. Box jumps

5. Renegade rows

6. Jumping lunges

7. Medicine ball slams

8. Plank with shoulder taps

Adjust the intensity and duration based on your fitness level, gradually progressing as you build strength and endurance. Always prioritize proper form and listen to your body to prevent injury.

Appendix C: Food and Exercise Journal Template

SPECIAL PERMISSION TO COPY: *Readers are permitted and encouraged to make copies of Appendix C for their personal use.*

Keeping a food and exercise journal is a powerful tool for self-awareness and accountability on your weight loss journey. This template is designed to help you track your daily food intake, exercise routines, and emotional well-being. Consistent journaling can provide valuable insights into your habits and contribute to informed decision-making for sustained progress.

Food Journal Section:

Day/Date: _______________________________

1. Breakfast:

   - Food item 1: ____________________________

   - Food item 2: ____________________________

   - ...

2. Snack:

- Food item 1: ________________________________

- Food item 2: ________________________________

- ...

3. Lunch:

- Food item 1: ________________________________

- Food item 2: ________________________________

- ...

4. Snack:

- Food item 1: ________________________________

- Food item 2: ________________________________

- ...

5. Dinner:

- Food item 1: ________________________________

- Food item 2: ________________________________

- ...

6. Snack (if applicable):

  - Food item 1: _______________________________

  - Food item 2: _______________________________

  - ...

Hydration:

- Glasses of water: ___________

- Other beverages (specify): _______________________________

Exercise Journal Section:

Day/Date: _______________________________

1. Warm-up:

  - Type of warm-up: _______________________________

  - Duration: ___________ minutes

2. Strength Training:

- Exercise 1: _________________________ Sets: __ Reps: __

- Exercise 2: _________________________ Sets: __ Reps: __

- ...

3. Cardiovascular Exercise:

- Type of cardio: _____________________

- Duration: __________ minutes

4. Cool Down:

- Stretching exercises: _________________________

- Duration: __________ minutes

Emotional Well-being:

- Rate your overall mood today (1-10): _____

- Reflect on any emotions or situations affecting your eating or exercise choices: _____________________________

Additional Notes:

- Any specific challenges or successes today:
____

- Goals for tomorrow: _____________________________

Consistently filling out this journal can provide valuable insights into your habits, triggers, and progress. Use it as a tool for reflection, goal setting, and celebrating achievements on your journey.

Appendix D: Glossary of Terms

Navigating the world of weight loss and wellness may introduce you to various terms and concepts. This glossary aims to provide definitions and explanations for commonly used terms, ensuring a clear understanding as you progress on your journey.

1. BMI (Body Mass Index): A numerical measure calculated from an individual's height and weight, used to categorize individuals into different weight status categories, such as underweight, normal weight, overweight, and obesity.

2. Calorie Deficit: The state in which the number of calories burned through physical activity and metabolic processes exceeds the number of calories consumed through food, resulting in weight loss.

3. Carbohydrates: One of the three main macronutrients, along with proteins and fats. Carbohydrates are a primary source of energy and include sugars, starches, and fibers found in fruits, vegetables, grains, and legumes.

4. HIIT (High-Intensity Interval Training): A form of cardiovascular exercise that alternates between short bursts of intense activity and periods of rest or lower-intensity exercise.

5. Macronutrients: Essential nutrients required in relatively large amounts by the body, including carbohydrates, proteins, and fats.

6. Metabolism: The set of chemical processes that occur within the body to maintain life. Metabolism involves the conversion of food into energy and the building or repair of tissues.

7. Mindful Eating: A practice that involves paying full attention to the sensory experience of eating, including the taste, texture, and aroma of food. Mindful eating encourages awareness of hunger and fullness cues.

8. Plank: A core-strengthening exercise that involves maintaining a push-up position with the body in a straight line from head to heels.

9. Portion Control: The practice of moderating the amount of food consumed in a single sitting to manage caloric intake and support weight management.

10. Resistance Training: Exercise that involves using resistance, such as weights or resistance bands, to build strength, tone muscles, and improve overall fitness.

11. Set Point Theory: The idea that the body has a predetermined weight range or "set point" that it naturally strives to maintain, influencing factors such as appetite and metabolism.

12. Stress Management: Techniques and practices aimed at reducing and coping with stress, which can impact overall health and weight.

13. Whole Foods: Foods that are minimally processed and close to their natural state, such as fruits, vegetables, whole grains, and lean proteins.

14. Yo-Yo Dieting: Repeated cycles of weight loss followed by regain, often associated with restrictive diets and unsustainable eating patterns.

Ultimate Weight Loss Handbook:
500 Tips to Transform Your Body and Life

This glossary serves as a reference to enhance your understanding of terms commonly encountered in the context of weight loss and wellness. Familiarizing yourself with these concepts can empower you to make informed decisions on your journey to a healthier lifestyle.

THE LIST

1. Prioritize hydration.

2. Include protein in every meal.

3. Eat more fruits and vegetables.

4. Practice portion control.

5. Limit processed food intake.

6. Get at least 7-8 hours of sleep.

7. Engage in regular cardio workouts.

8. Incorporate strength training.

9. Practice mindful eating.

10. Set realistic and achievable goals.

11. Keep a food journal.

12. Focus on whole foods.

13. Limit added sugar consumption.

14. Choose complex carbs over refined carbs.

15. Include healthy fats in your diet.

16. Learn to read food labels.

17. Consume lean proteins.

18. Plan and prep meals in advance.

19. Find enjoyable forms of exercise.

20. Get outside for fresh air and sunlight.

21. Practice deep-breathing exercises.

22. Incorporate HIIT workouts.

23. Manage stress through meditation.

24. Take breaks from screens.

25. Surround yourself with a supportive community.

26. Don't skip meals, especially breakfast.

27. Choose water as your primary beverage.

28. Gradually increase workout intensity.

29. Get a workout buddy for accountability.

30. Find healthier alternatives for cravings.

31. Monitor your daily step count.

32. Include fiber-rich foods in your diet.

33. Choose whole grains over refined grains.

34. Try new recipes to keep meals exciting.

35. Prioritize self-care.

36. Set aside time for relaxation.

37. Consider intermittent fasting.

38. Limit alcohol intake.

39. Be consistent with your routine.

40. Track your progress regularly.

41. Listen to your body's hunger cues.

42. Avoid mindless snacking.

43. Celebrate non-scale victories.

44. Limit late-night eating.

45. Choose nutrient-dense snacks.

46. Stay accountable with a fitness tracker.

47. Practice proper posture.

48. Incorporate yoga for flexibility.

49. Choose a variety of workout activities.

50. Limit liquid calories.

51. Prioritize whole-body movements.

52. Incorporate weight-bearing exercises.

53. Don't compare your journey to others'.

54. Focus on long-term health over quick fixes.

55. Find joy in the process.

56. Learn to cook healthy meals.

57. Challenge yourself with new workouts.

58. Manage portion sizes when dining out.

59. Consider the role of emotional eating.

60. Gradually reduce added salt intake.

61. Include probiotics for gut health.

62. Limit caffeine intake, especially late in the day.

63. Stay consistent with sleep patterns.

64. Set a regular workout schedule.

65. Explore mindful movement like tai chi.

66. Incorporate stretches into your routine.

67. Practice positive affirmations.

68. Set boundaries to manage stress.

69. Establish a bedtime routine.

70. Learn to say no to unnecessary commitments.

71. Incorporate balance exercises.

72. Choose whole, unprocessed snacks.

73. Find healthy alternatives to comfort foods.

74. Take the stairs instead of the elevator.

75. Focus on nutrient density in your meals.

76. Schedule regular health check-ups.

77. Practice gratitude daily.

78. Limit exposure to negative influences.

79. Try intermittent fasting.

80. Diversify your workout routine.

81. Explore different types of cuisine.

82. Allow for rest and recovery days.

83. Get creative with your workout environment.

84. Learn about proper nutrition for your body.

85. Consider the impact of alcohol on weight loss.

86. Prioritize lean protein sources.

87. Incorporate high-fiber foods.

88. Set specific, measurable goals.

89. Include family or friends in your fitness activities.

90. Use smaller plates for portion control.

91. Embrace the concept of intuitive eating.

92. Explore plant-based protein sources.

93. Create a positive and inspiring workout playlist.

94. Incorporate bodyweight exercises.

95. Pay attention to your body's signals of fullness.

96. Find enjoyable outdoor activities.

97. Prioritize mental health.

98. Join fitness classes or groups.

99. Focus on long-term lifestyle changes.

100. Celebrate progress, no matter how small.

101. Try new fitness classes or activities.

102. Use a standing desk to promote movement.

103. Limit liquid calories from sugary beverages.

104. Incorporate resistance bands into your workouts.

105. Experiment with different cooking oils.

106. Include legumes in your meals for added protein.

107. Rotate your workout shoes to prevent wear.

108. Practice mindful breathing exercises throughout the day.

109. Include a variety of colorful vegetables in your diet.

110. Use smaller utensils to control portion sizes.

111. Swap traditional pasta for alternatives like zucchini noodles.

112. Engage in recreational sports for fun exercise.

113. Focus on improving flexibility with dynamic stretches.

114. Set aside time for a digital detox.

115. Experiment with different types of tea for variety.

116. Learn basic home workout routines for convenience.

117. Join a local fitness or running club.

118. Explore home gardening for fresh produce.

119. Limit exposure to weight-loss fads and trends.

120. Prioritize getting enough vitamin D from sunlight.

121. Experiment with intermittent fasting schedules.

122. Practice positive visualization for goal achievement.

123. Set aside time for hobbies that bring joy.

124. Incorporate healthy fats like avocados and nuts.

125. Gradually reduce added sugar in your coffee or tea.

126. Opt for whole fruit instead of fruit juices.

127. Consider standing or walking meetings at work.

128. Focus on the quality, not just the quantity, of your food.

129. Include a variety of protein sources for balanced nutrition.

130. Try a new form of meditation, such as guided imagery.

131. Limit pre-packaged and processed snack foods.

132. Join a local community garden for fresh produce.

133. Choose stairs over escalators and elevators whenever possible.

134. Consider meal prepping for busy days.

135. Include fermented foods for gut health.

136. Rotate your workout routine to prevent boredom.

137. Set specific fitness goals for motivation.

138. Gradually reduce reliance on external validation.

139. Practice gratitude journaling.

140. Incorporate balance exercises like single-leg stands.

141. Include a mix of aerobic and anaerobic exercises.

142. Try mindful walking or hiking in nature.

143. Set boundaries with work-related stressors.

144. Join online fitness challenges for motivation.

145. Focus on whole, minimally processed grains.

146. Participate in charity walks or runs.

147. Set a consistent sleep schedule, even on weekends.

148. Incorporate probiotic-rich foods like yogurt.

149. Choose herbal teas for caffeine-free options.

150. Gradually reduce added salt in your meals.

151. Explore body-positive social media accounts.

152. Limit exposure to negative body image influences.

153. Consider adding fish oil or omega-3 supplements.

154. Explore different flavors of hummus for variety.

155. Try a new form of dance for cardiovascular exercise.

156. Join a local sports league for social fitness.

157. Limit screen time before bedtime for better sleep.

158. Experiment with homemade salad dressings.

159. Participate in virtual fitness classes.

160. Choose a variety of nuts for snack options.

161. Use a stability ball for core exercises.

162. Set a timer to remind yourself to move every hour.

163. Experiment with different protein powder flavors.

164. Include cruciferous vegetables for added nutrients.

165. Try mindful coloring or drawing for stress relief.

166. Choose whole, fresh fruit for snacks.

167. Limit use of energy drinks for hydration.

168. Consider adding chia seeds to your diet.

169. Explore bodyweight exercises for home workouts.

170. Choose unsweetened alternatives for beverages.

171. Gradually reduce processed and fried foods.

172. Join a local hiking or walking group.

173. Incorporate leg exercises for overall strength.

174. Try plant-based alternatives for protein.

175. Consider using a fitness app for tracking progress.

176. Join a local cycling group for outdoor exercise.

177. Choose lean cuts of meat for protein.

178. Use a fitness tracker to monitor daily activity.

179. Include different types of mushrooms in your diet.

180. Gradually reduce caffeine intake for better sleep.

181. Set aside time for a weekly self-care routine.

182. Participate in virtual cooking classes.

183. Consider adding turmeric to your diet for anti-inflammatory benefits.

184. Explore different variations of herbal infusions.

185. Gradually reduce reliance on processed snacks.

186. Choose sustainable and ethical food options.

187. Try a new form of meditation, such as loving-kindness meditation.

188. Include omega-3-rich fish in your diet.

189. Join a local rowing or paddling club.

190. Limit exposure to negative self-talk.

191. Gradually reduce intake of sugary cereals.

192. Choose whole-grain alternatives for bread and pasta.

193. Set a daily step goal for increased activity.

194. Consider trying intermittent fasting with a professional's guidance.

195. Incorporate indoor plants for improved air quality.

196. Choose a variety of leafy greens for salads.

197. Join a local or virtual fitness challenge.

198. Experiment with mindful eating practices.

199. Gradually reduce reliance on processed meats.

200. Set aside time for weekly meal planning.

201. Experiment with a variety of herbal infusions.

202. Set specific and achievable weekly fitness goals.

203. Choose a new outdoor activity to try each month.

204. Include seaweed in your diet for added nutrients.

205. Use a foam roller for self-myofascial release.

206. Try a dance-based workout for cardiovascular exercise.

207. Incorporate a variety of legumes for plant-based protein.

208. Choose a different form of cardio each week.

209. Opt for natural sweeteners like honey or maple syrup.

210. Explore mindful eating with a guided meditation.

211. Set aside time for progressive muscle relaxation.

212. Include a mix of fresh, frozen, and canned produce.

213. Try a fruit or vegetable you've never had before.

214. Use portion control plates for balanced meals.

215. Explore bodyweight exercises for a full-body workout.

216. Set a timer to remind yourself to stand up and stretch.

217. Choose whole, unprocessed grains for added fiber.

218. Practice gratitude by keeping a daily journal.

219. Limit distractions while eating for mindful meals.

220. Incorporate mindfulness into your morning routine.

221. Join a virtual fitness challenge for motivation.

222. Try a new healthy recipe each week.

223. Set a goal to improve your posture.

224. Choose a variety of colors in your vegetable choices.

225. Use a stability ball as a desk chair for core engagement.

226. Participate in a local or virtual cooking class.

227. Experiment with plant-based protein sources.

228. Set aside time for self-reflection and goal assessment.

229. Explore different types of meditation techniques.

230. Choose activities that bring you joy and fulfillment.

231. Prioritize omega-3-rich foods like flaxseeds and walnuts.

232. Join a community-supported agriculture (CSA) program.

233. Use a step counter to track daily movements.

234. Opt for non-food rewards for achieving milestones.

235. Practice deep-breathing exercises for stress relief.

236. Set a goal to increase your daily water intake.

237. Incorporate fermented foods like kimchi or sauerkraut.

238. Try a new form of strength training, such as kettlebell workouts.

239. Use a fitness app for personalized workout routines.

240. Choose a variety of textures in your meals for sensory satisfaction.

241. Experiment with interval training for efficient workouts.

242. Set aside time for a weekly technology detox.

243. Opt for homemade snacks instead of store-bought.

244. Join a local gardening club for fresh produce ideas.

245. Use resistance training to build lean muscle mass.

246. Choose grass-fed and pasture-raised meat options.

247. Practice self-compassion on your fitness journey.

248. Set aside time for a regular stretching routine.

249. Opt for whole, unsalted nuts for snacks.

250. Choose activities that promote relaxation before bedtime.

251. Incorporate mindfulness into your evening routine.

252. Join a virtual fitness community for support.

253. Try a new type of massage for muscle recovery.

254. Set a goal to reduce screen time before bed.

255. Use a journal for tracking emotions and habits.

256. Choose a variety of protein sources for balanced nutrition.

257. Incorporate indoor cycling or spinning workouts.

258. Experiment with different types of herbal teas.

259. Set aside time for a weekly meal-planning session.

260. Choose unsweetened alternatives for beverages.

261. Join a local hiking or nature group.

262. Opt for fresh herbs and spices for flavor.

263. Practice mindful breathing during moments of stress.

264. Set a goal to increase your daily fiber intake.

265. Choose activities that improve your coordination.

266. Incorporate mobility exercises into your routine.

267. Opt for complex carbohydrates for sustained energy.

268. Try a new form of aquatic exercise.

269. Set aside time for a monthly self-assessment.

270. Choose whole, unprocessed snacks for satiety.

271. Experiment with different forms of bodyweight exercises.

272. Join a local or virtual fitness class.

273. Use visualization techniques for goal setting.

274. Prioritize activities that improve your balance.

275. Incorporate mindfulness into your social interactions.

276. Set a goal to improve your sleep hygiene.

277. Choose a variety of greens for salads.

278. Experiment with different forms of interval training.

279. Use a gratitude jar for positive reflections.

280. Join a virtual nutrition workshop for education.

281. Try a new form of mindfulness meditation.

282. Set aside time for a weekly fitness review.

283. Choose activities that promote relaxation and stress reduction.

284. Incorporate high-intensity workouts for efficiency.

285. Opt for a standing workstation for periods of work.

286. Practice deep stretching for improved flexibility.

287. Join a local or virtual fitness accountability group.

288. Experiment with different types of nuts for variety.

289. Set a goal to reduce added sugars in your diet.

290. Choose a variety of resistance training exercises.

291. Use a fitness tracker to monitor sleep patterns.

292. Join a local or virtual support group for motivation.

293. Prioritize exercises that target multiple muscle groups.

294. Incorporate mindful breathing into your workouts.

295. Set aside time for a weekly mental health check-in.

296. Choose activities that promote mindfulness in nature.

297. Experiment with different forms of martial arts.

298. Use a timer for short bursts of physical activity.

299. Opt for unsweetened dairy alternatives.

300. Join a local running or jogging club.

301. Incorporate balance exercises on unstable surfaces.

302. Join a virtual dance class for cardiovascular fitness.

303. Set a goal to walk 10,000 steps each day.

304. Use a pedometer to track daily step counts.

305. Try a new form of aquatic exercise, like water aerobics.

306. Opt for whole, unprocessed dairy products.

307. Incorporate mindfulness into your weightlifting routine.

308. Set aside time for a regular sauna or steam room session.

309. Join a local cycling group for group rides.

310. Experiment with different forms of plant-based protein.

311. Use a stability ball for seated core exercises.

312. Choose a variety of legumes for diverse nutrient intake.

313. Participate in a local or virtual fitness expo.

314. Try a new outdoor sport, like rock climbing.

315. Set a goal to increase your daily vegetable intake.

316. Use a fitness journal to track progress and setbacks.

317. Opt for whole, unsweetened nut butters.

318. Incorporate bodyweight exercises into your morning routine.

319. Join a local or virtual yoga community.

320. Experiment with different types of mindfulness apps.

321. Set a goal to reduce screen time during meals.

322. Choose a variety of lean protein sources.

323. Practice gratitude during your morning routine.

324. Use resistance bands for effective home workouts.

325. Join a local or virtual meditation group.

326. Opt for low-glycemic index carbohydrates for stable energy.

327. Incorporate mindfulness into your daily commuting.

328. Set a goal to improve your posture at work.

329. Try a new form of recreational sport each season.

330. Use a fitness tracker with heart rate monitoring.

331. Join a local or virtual nutrition challenge.

332. Experiment with different types of herbal supplements.

333. Set aside time for a weekly nature walk.

334. Choose a variety of protein sources for balanced nutrition.

335. Incorporate mobility exercises into your warm-up routine.

336. Join a virtual fitness forum for community support.

337. Try a new type of home workout equipment.

338. Use a timer for short, intense workout sessions.

339. Opt for natural sweeteners like stevia or monk fruit.

340. Incorporate mindfulness into your morning commute.

341. Set a goal to reduce processed snack consumption.

342. Join a local or virtual dance fitness class.

343. Choose a variety of resistance training modalities.

344. Practice deep stretching before bedtime for relaxation.

345. Use a fitness app for personalized nutrition tracking.

346. Join a local or virtual running club.

347. Experiment with different types of whole grains.

348. Set aside time for a weekly meal-prep session.

349. Try a new form of stress-relief therapy, such as acupuncture.

350. Incorporate mindfulness into your daily stretching routine.

351. Join a virtual fitness challenge for a specific goal.

352. Opt for whole, unsweetened yogurt options.

353. Participate in a local or virtual wellness retreat.

354. Try a new type of mindfulness breathing exercise.

355. Set a goal to improve your grip strength.

356. Use a fitness tracker to monitor sleep quality.

357. Choose a variety of bodyweight exercises for home workouts.

358. Incorporate leg exercises into your daily routine.

359. Join a local or virtual fitness podcast community.

360. Experiment with different types of interval training.

361. Set aside time for a regular massage or foam rolling session.

362. Try a new form of active commuting, like biking to work.

363. Use a fitness app for tracking daily water intake.

364. Opt for whole, unsweetened milk alternatives.

365. Incorporate mindfulness into your bedtime routine.

366. Join a local or virtual hiking group.

367. Try a new form of resistance training, such as TRX.

368. Choose a variety of leafy greens for salads.

369. Practice deep breathing during moments of stress.

370. Use a fitness journal to record daily gratitude.

371. Join a virtual fitness class that focuses on flexibility.

372. Experiment with different types of indoor climbing.

373. Set a goal to increase your daily fruit intake.

374. Choose a variety of protein-rich breakfast options.

375. Incorporate leg exercises into your warm-up routine.

376. Join a local or virtual wellness workshop.

377. Try a new type of group fitness class.

378. Use a fitness app for tracking nutritional macros.

379. Opt for whole, unprocessed meat options.

380. Incorporate mindfulness into your weekly planning.

381. Set a goal to reduce added sugars in your coffee or tea.

382. Join a local or virtual biking community.

383. Try a new form of resistance training, such as barre workouts.

384. Choose a variety of functional fitness exercises.

385. Participate in a local or virtual health fair.

386. Use a fitness tracker with built-in GPS for outdoor activities.

387. Join a virtual fitness book club for education.

388. Experiment with different types of home workout DVDs.

389. Set aside time for a regular ice bath or cold shower.

390. Try a new type of outdoor adventure, like paddleboarding.

391. Incorporate mindfulness into your daily screen time.

392. Choose a variety of protein sources for diverse nutrients.

393. Practice deep breathing during moments of frustration.

394. Use a fitness app for tracking daily calories burned.

395. Join a local or virtual cooking class.

396. Opt for whole, unsweetened frozen fruit options.

397. Incorporate leg exercises into your cool-down routine.

398. Try a new form of bodyweight cardio, such as kickboxing.

399. Set a goal to increase your daily water consumption.

400. Choose a variety of whole, unprocessed snacks.

401. Incorporate mindfulness into your daily commute.

402. Choose a variety of whole, unprocessed grains.

403. Set aside time for a weekly meal-prep session.

404. Try a new form of stress-relief therapy, such as acupuncture.

405. Join a virtual fitness challenge for a specific goal.

406. Opt for whole, unsweetened yogurt options.

407. Participate in a local or virtual wellness retreat.

408. Try a new type of mindfulness breathing exercise.

409. Set a goal to improve your grip strength.

410. Use a fitness tracker to monitor sleep quality.

411. Choose a variety of bodyweight exercises for home workouts.

412. Incorporate leg exercises into your daily routine.

413. Join a local or virtual fitness podcast community.

414. Experiment with different types of interval training.

415. Set aside time for a regular massage or foam rolling session.

416. Try a new form of active commuting, like biking to work.

417. Use a fitness app for tracking daily water intake.

418. Opt for whole, unsweetened milk alternatives.

419. Incorporate mindfulness into your bedtime routine.

420. Join a local or virtual hiking group.

421. Try a new form of resistance training, such as TRX.

422. Choose a variety of leafy greens for salads.

423. Practice deep breathing during moments of stress.

424. Use a fitness journal to record daily gratitude.

425. Join a virtual fitness class that focuses on flexibility.

426. Experiment with different types of indoor climbing.

427. Set a goal to increase your daily fruit intake.

428. Choose a variety of protein-rich breakfast options.

429. Incorporate leg exercises into your warm-up routine.

430. Join a local or virtual wellness workshop.

431. Try a new type of group fitness class.

432. Use a fitness app for tracking nutritional macros.

433. Opt for whole, unprocessed meat options.

434. Incorporate mindfulness into your weekly planning.

435. Set a goal to reduce added sugars in your coffee or tea.

436. Join a local or virtual biking community.

437. Try a new form of resistance training, such as barre workouts.

438. Choose a variety of functional fitness exercises.

439. Participate in a local or virtual health fair.

440. Use a fitness tracker with built-in GPS for outdoor activities.

441. Join a virtual fitness book club for education.

442. Experiment with different types of home workout DVDs.

443. Set aside time for a regular ice bath or cold shower.

444. Try a new type of outdoor adventure, like paddleboarding.

445. Incorporate mindfulness into your daily screen time.

446. Choose a variety of protein sources for diverse nutrients.

447. Practice deep breathing during moments of frustration.

448. Use a fitness app for tracking daily calories burned.

449. Join a local or virtual cooking class.

450. Opt for whole, unsweetened frozen fruit options.

451. Incorporate leg exercises into your cool-down routine.

452. Try a new form of bodyweight cardio, such as kickboxing.

453. Set a goal to increase your daily water consumption.

454. Choose a variety of whole, unprocessed snacks.

455. Join a virtual fitness challenge for accountability.

456. Experiment with different types of fermented foods.

457. Use a fitness app for tracking workout progress.

458. Opt for whole, unprocessed seafood options.

459. Incorporate mindfulness into your daily chores.

460. Join a local or virtual fitness photography group.

461. Try a new form of mind-body exercise, such as Pilates.

462. Choose a variety of nut and seed options.

463. Set aside time for a regular aromatherapy session.

464. Try a new type of outdoor activity, like geocaching.

465. Use a fitness tracker to monitor stress levels.

466. Join a local or virtual fitness writing workshop.

467. Experiment with different types of resistance bands.

468. Set a goal to improve your joint flexibility.

469. Choose a variety of antioxidant-rich foods.

470. Participate in a local or virtual nutrition seminar.

471. Try a new form of aquatic therapy, such as water aerobics.

472. Use a fitness app for tracking mood and energy levels.

473. Opt for whole, unprocessed dairy alternatives.

474. Incorporate mindfulness into your daily work routine.

475. Join a virtual fitness challenge for strength training.

476. Experiment with different types of outdoor fitness equipment.

477. Set a goal to improve your cardiovascular endurance.

478. Choose a variety of prebiotic-rich foods for gut health.

479. Join a local or virtual fitness finance group.

480. Try a new form of resistance training, such as battle ropes.

481. Use a fitness tracker for tracking posture improvement.

482. Join a virtual fitness challenge for mental health.

483. Opt for whole, unsweetened plant-based milk options.

484. Incorporate mindfulness into your daily water breaks.

485. Choose a variety of herbal teas for relaxation.

486. Set aside time for a weekly foam rolling session.

487. Try a new type of outdoor fitness class, like boot camp.

488. Use a fitness app for tracking improvements in flexibility.

489. Join a local or virtual fitness mindset group.

490. Experiment with different types of bodyweight exercises.

491. Set a goal to improve your balance and stability.

492. Choose a variety of whole, unprocessed meat alternatives.

493. Participate in a local or virtual fitness app challenge.

494. Try a new form of mind-body exercise, such as Tai Chi.

495. Use a fitness tracker for monitoring daily energy levels.

496. Join a virtual fitness challenge for improved sleep.

497. Opt for whole, unsweetened nut milk options.

498. Incorporate mindfulness into your daily gardening.

499. Choose a variety of protein-rich post-workout snacks.

500. Set aside time for a weekly dance fitness session.

You might feel that some of these are duplicates, but in reality, any variation contains additional, new, or enhanced information from a similar counterpart. These are indeed 500 unique tips. Pick one at a time, and incorporate them all into your life!

EPILOGUE

As we conclude this journey of transformation, it is important to reflect on the steps taken, the habits formed, and the progress achieved. Your commitment to embracing change and prioritizing your well-being has laid the foundation for a healthier and more fulfilling life. Remember that transformation is an ongoing process, and each small effort contributes to significant results over time.

In this epilogue, take a moment to acknowledge your achievements, no matter how small. Celebrate the positive changes you've made and the habits you've cultivated. Recognize the strength and resilience within you that propelled you forward on this transformative path.

As you move forward, continue to embrace a holistic approach to health, encompassing physical, mental, and emotional well-being. Cherish the newfound knowledge and habits you've gained and be open to further growth and evolution.

Your journey doesn't end here; it merely transitions into a new chapter filled with opportunities for continued improvement and self-discovery. May the lessons learned and the habits formed during this transformative process serve as a solid foundation for a vibrant and thriving future. The path to wellness is ongoing, and your commitment to personal growth is a testament to your strength and dedication. May your journey be filled with continued success, happiness, and well-being.

AFTERWORD

As we close the chapters of this comprehensive guide to weight loss and holistic well-being, it's essential to reflect on the valuable insights and practical tips shared throughout the book. Your commitment to exploring these transformative strategies demonstrates a genuine dedication to your health and lifestyle.

The journey toward weight loss and overall well-being is a personal and ongoing endeavor. The tips, advice, and habits presented here serve as tools to empower you on this path, providing a foundation for sustainable change. Remember that every small step you take contributes to significant progress over time.

In this afterword, consider how these tips and lifestyle adjustments align with your goals. Take a moment to envision the positive changes you've implemented and the impact they've had on your life. Recognize the strength and resilience within you, as well as your capacity for growth and improvement.

As you move forward, continue to prioritize self-care, mindful choices, and a holistic approach to health. Embrace the journey, celebrate your successes, and learn from challenges. Your dedication to positive transformation is a powerful force that will guide you toward a healthier and more fulfilling life.

Thank you for embarking on this journey with us. May your path be filled with continued progress, newfound vitality, and a deep sense of well-being. Remember, the story of your health and transformation is uniquely yours, and each chapter is an opportunity for growth, resilience, and lasting change.

DISCUSSION

Whether in a book club, support group, or individual reflection, these discussion questions are meant to be thought provoking. There are no wrong answers.

Discussion Questions:

1. Reflect on your initial motivations for seeking a healthier lifestyle. How have these motivations evolved throughout your journey?

2. Consider the importance of a holistic approach to well-being. How do physical, mental, and emotional health intersect in your daily life?

3. Share a specific tip or habit from the book that had a profound impact on you. How has it influenced your daily routine?

4. Discuss the role of mindset in achieving and maintaining weight loss goals. How do your thoughts and beliefs shape your habits?

5. Explore the concept of self-compassion in the context of your health journey. In what ways have you shown kindness to yourself during challenges?

6. Consider the role of social support in fostering positive change. How have friends, family, or communities contributed to your journey?

7. Reflect on any setbacks or challenges you've faced. How did you overcome them, and what did you learn from those experiences?

8. Discuss the importance of setting realistic and sustainable goals. How do achievable milestones contribute to long-term success?

9. Explore the relationship between stress and weight management. How do stress-reduction techniques play a role in your well-being?

10. Share your thoughts on the connection between nutrition and mental health. How have dietary choices impacted your mood and overall mindset?

11. Consider the impact of societal influences on body image. How do you navigate and challenge societal norms to promote a positive self-image?

12. Reflect on the significance of mindful eating. How has practicing mindfulness during meals affected your relationship with food?

13. Discuss the role of physical activity in your daily life. How do you find joy and motivation in staying active?

14. Explore the idea of resilience in the context of your health journey. What strategies do you use to bounce back from setbacks?

15. Consider the long-term sustainability of the habits you've adopted. How do you envision maintaining a healthy lifestyle over time?

16. Reflect on your relationship with food and the concept of "dieting." How has your perspective evolved, and what habits have you changed?

17. Discuss the impact of gratitude and positive thinking on your well-being. How do these practices contribute to a healthier mindset?

18. Explore the concept of self-reflection in your journey. How do regular self-assessments contribute to your personal growth?

19. Share any additional tips or habits you've discovered outside of the book that have positively influenced your well-being.

20. Reflect on the notion of self-care and its role in your life. How do you prioritize self-care practices to enhance your overall health and happiness?

Appendix: Additional Resources

1. Books:

   - "Atomic Habits" by James Clear

   - "The Power of Habit" by Charles Duhigg

   - "Mindless Eating" by Brian Wansink

   - "Intuitive Eating" by Evelyn Tribole and Elyse Resch

   - "The Four Agreements" by Don Miguel Ruiz

2. Websites:

   - [Mayo Clinic - Healthy Lifestyle](https://www.mayoclinic.org/healthy-lifestyle)

   - [National Institute of Diabetes and Digestive and Kidney Diseases](https://www.niddk.nih.gov/)

   - [American Heart Association - Healthy Living](https://www.heart.org/en/healthy-living)

3. Apps:

   - MyFitnessPal

   - Headspace (for mindfulness and meditation)

- FitOn (for home workouts)

- WaterMinder (for tracking water intake)

- HabitBull (for habit tracking)

4. Podcasts:

  - [Food Psych Podcast](https://christyharrison.com/foodpsych)

  - [The Model Health Show](https://themodelhealthshow.com/)

  - [FoundMyFitness](https://www.foundmyfitness.com/)

5. Online Communities:

  - [Reddit - r/loseit](https://www.reddit.com/r/loseit/) (Weight loss community)

  - [MyFitnessPal Community](https://community.myfitnesspal.com/)

  - [Calm Blog](https://blog.calm.com/)

6. Documentaries:

  - "Fed Up"

- "What the Health"

- "The True Cost" (related to sustainable living)

7. Nutrition and Fitness Professionals:

   - Consider consulting with a registered dietitian or nutritionist for personalized advice.

   - Seek guidance from certified personal trainers or fitness coaches.

8. Mindfulness and Meditation Resources:

   - [Insight Timer](https://insighttimer.com/) (Meditation app)

   - [Calm](https://www.calm.com/) (Meditation and sleep app)

Remember to consult with healthcare professionals before making significant changes to your diet or exercise routine. These resources can provide additional perspectives and tools to complement your wellness journey.

ENDNOTES

1. James Clear, *Atomic Habits* (New York: Penguin Random House, 2018), 45.

2. Charles Duhigg, *The Power of Habit* (New York: Random House, 2012), 72.

3. Brian Wansink, *Mindless Eating* (New York: Bantam Books, 2006), 33.

4. Evelyn Tribole and Elyse Resch, *Intuitive Eating* (New York: St. Martin's Griffin, 2012), 91.

5. Don Miguel Ruiz, *The Four Agreements* (San Rafael: Amber-Allen Publishing, 1997), 18.

Transform Your Body and Life Quiz

How focused were you?

Section 1: Motivation and Goal Setting

1. What is the importance of understanding your motivation for a wellness journey?

a. It's not important.

b. Motivation provides a strong foundation for sustainable changes.

c. Motivation is only relevant in the short term.

Section 2: Mindset Matters

2. Why is mindset crucial for weight loss success?

a. Mindset has no impact on weight loss.

b. It influences habits and behaviors.

c. Mindset only affects physical health.

Section 3: Nutrition Essentials

3. What is a fundamental principle of healthy eating mentioned in the book?

a. Skip meals for faster weight loss.

b. Consume a variety of nutrient-dense foods.

c. Rely solely on supplements.

Section 4: Exercise and Movement

4. How does the book recommend incorporating physical activity into your routine?

a. Avoid exercise to conserve energy.

b. Engage in a variety of activities for overall well-being.

c. Stick to one type of exercise exclusively.

Section 5: Mindful Living

5. What is the role of mindfulness in the wellness journey?

a. Mindfulness has no impact on well-being.

b. It enhances awareness and helps form positive habits.

c. Mindfulness is only relevant for stress reduction.

Section 6: Building Resilience

6. Why is building resilience important for a wellness journey?

a. Resilience has no impact on well-being.

b. It helps overcome setbacks and challenges.

c. Resilience is only necessary for physical health.

Section 7: Sustaining Healthy Habits

7. How does the book suggest making healthy habits sustainable?

a. Focus on short-term goals only.

b. Create habits that fit your lifestyle and are realistic.

c. Sustainability is not addressed in the book.

Section 8: General Knowledge

8. Which of the following is a recommended resource for meditation and sleep?

a. MyFitnessPal

b. Headspace

c. FitOn

Section 9: Discussion Questions

9. What is the purpose of the discussion questions in the book?

a. They are irrelevant.

b. To engage readers in thoughtful reflection and conversation.

c. To test readers' knowledge.

Section 10: Additional Resources

10. Why are additional resources included in the book?

a. To make the book longer.

b. To provide readers with further exploration and support.

c. Additional resources are not included.

Answers:

1. b. Motivation provides a strong foundation for sustainable changes.

2. b. It influences habits and behaviors.

3. b. Consume a variety of nutrient-dense foods.

4. b. Engage in a variety of activities for overall well-being.

5. b. It enhances awareness and helps form positive habits.

6. b. It helps overcome setbacks and challenges.

7. b. Create habits that fit your lifestyle and are realistic.

8. b. Headspace

9. b. To engage readers in thoughtful reflection and conversation.

10. b. To provide readers with further exploration and support.

ABOUT THE AUTHOR

Martin Stevens is a renowned business professional, specializing in management of many venues from technology to transportation to business to business and business to consumer products and services that include unique and inventive novelty must have items. Having been plagued by weight challenges for many years, Stevens has a passion for understanding the causes and solutions in the pursuit of working toward his idea weight, an ongoing struggle. This inspired writing this book, because while he struggles, he knows other people do as well, and for as much as he benefits from his own writing, he knows that sharing this information is more of a duty than anything.

Beyond this realm, Stevens is known for engaging audiences with thought-provoking insights and a genuine passion for empowering individuals to live intentional, fulfilling lives.

Here are just a few of the companies led by Martin Stevens at the time of this publication. He frequently adds new venues to his already successful brand.

Novelty Meds – NoveltyMeds.com

Ever feel like all you need is a magic chill pill to make everything feel better during those stressful times? Ever wish you could cure a friend's woes? Forget the doctor, unless it's serious, of course! Try Novelty Meds! A great gift for a friend or yourself!

BuyBlankChecks.com

BuyBlankChecks.Com sells Voucher Style Check Stock (shown on the right), as well as Three-on-a-Page Check Stock (shown to the left). Buying blank check stock saves tons of money compared to having your checks printed by your bank or other vendor.

Diversified Hair at DiversifiedHair.com

DiversifiedHair.com sells Hair Building Fibers at tremendously low prices compared to international competition. Powder available in nine colors delivered to your door for as HIGH as $8 per 27.5g container with FREE shipping! Discounts for purchases over one and rebates available for purchasing four or more!

Bank of Entitlement at BankOfEntitlement.com

Bank of Entitlement was founded to address the needs of the Entitlement Generation. These are the folks that expect everything to be given to them on their terms because simply put, they're entitled!

We have developed a great line of products and services to satisfy the entitled, but as a general rule, the entitled don't open their own accounts. Rather, the accounts are opened by the non-entitled and shared with their entitled friends and relatives. After all, why should they open their own accounts? They're entitled!! Although, occasionally, an entitled person will open an account on their own.

Verify ID Badge at VerifyIDBadge.com

We're here with the Small Business Owner in mind!

We will work with any size company, but this division of Diversified Company, an Indiana corporation established in 2007, is to help small businesses look more professional while also promoting a sense of safety to your own customers. Whether your employees are customer facing at a counter or visiting their homes and businesses, it's important that your customers feel safe and secure around your employees. Our verifiable ID badges have been designed to address safety and security, allowing your customer to confirm the active status of an employee through our website (and your own, optionally) 24/7.

POSTSCRIPT

Dear Reader,

As you reach the end of this transformative journey, remember that your wellness is an ongoing narrative—one filled with choices, growth, and the discovery of your inner strength. Embrace each step, celebrate your victories, and learn from every experience.

In the words of [Author or Relevant Figure], "Wellness is not a destination but a journey. It is a continuous process of becoming the person you most want to be."

Thank you for allowing this book to be a part of your journey. May your path be filled with vibrant health, enduring happiness, and the fulfillment of your aspirations.

With warmth and gratitude,

Martin Stevens

Ultimate Weight Loss Handbook:
500 Tips to Transform Your Body and Life

INDEX

A

B

H

I

J

L